INTRODUCTION

The importance of health and wellness has certainly come to the forefront of the health industry in the last decade. With the baby boomer generation nearing or entering their senior years, strained health and medical services, and the realization by greater numbers of people of the limitations of medical science, society has developed an increasingly prominent attitude of responsibility towards one's own health and wellness.

No longer are people solely relying on doctors or hospitals to make them better if they get sick. Instead, the approach has changed to one of illness prevention, to maintain or improve the state of health that already exists. The incredible boom in the health industry overall bears witness to these trends.

The importance of health and wellness is reflected by the fact that diets, weight loss programs, exercise programs and equipment, fitness facilities, spas, nutritional supplements and activity/leisure groups of all sorts are now commonplace in our everyday lives. Some of these changes are driven by the extreme demands and long waits for treatment in the health care system, but also by the desire of the working generation for a more active lifestyle after retirement, with the hope of being fit and well enough to participate in their chosen activities. For these goals to manifest into reality the base of good health must be built up throughout life, not just to try to repair the damage after it's been done.

So, it has become clear why the health industry has turned in its present direction. Only by placing the importance of health and wellness as a priority now can anyone make the most of their future.

The driving factors behind the drifts in health and wellness were attributed to the rate at which obesity is increasing across the globe. High rates of heart disease, cancer and various food-related diseases were growing at astronomical rates. These gory tales eventually drawn the attention of people to the needs for a healthy lifestyle, this discovery was matched with a series of corresponding researches and a lot of things were revealed about human anatomy and its associated health risks.

Therefore, health and wellness can be said to be a multidimensional issue because it can be attributed to the totality of human existence. It involves making conscious efforts to improve personal general state of health

Disclaimer

This book is geared towards providing exact and reliable information in regards to the topic and issues covered. The publication is sold on the idea that the publisher is not re□uired to render accounting, officially permitted, or otherwise, □ualified services. If advice is necessary, legal or professional, a practiced individual in the profession should be ordered.

From a Declaration of Principles which was accepted and approved e□ually by a Committee of the American Bar Association and a Committee of Publishers and Associations.

In no way is, it legal to reproduce, duplicate, or transmit any part of this document by either electronic means or in printed format. Recording of this publication is strictly prohibited and any storage of this document is not allowed unless with written permission from the publisher. All rights reserved.

The information provided herein is stated to be truthful and consistent, in that any liability, in terms of inattention or otherwise, by any usage or abuse of any policies, processes, or directions contained within is the solitary and utter responsibility of the recipient reader. Under no circumstances will any legal responsibility or blame be held against the publisher for any reparation, damages, or monetary loss due to the information herein, either directly or indirectly.

Respective authors own all copyrights not held by the publisher.

INTRODUCTION   1

Disclaimer   3

CHAPTER ONE   7

INTRODUCTION TO HEALTH AND WELLNESS   7

WHAT IS HEALTH AND WELLNESS?   8

IMPORTANCE OF HEALTH AND WELLNESS   13

FOUR PILLARS OF HEALTH AND WELLNESS   16

SETTING GOALS TO ACHIEVE IMPROVED HEALTH AND
WELLNESS   20

LAW OF ATTRACTION- HOW THE LAW OF ATTRACTION
SUPPORTS HEALTH AND WELLNESS   25

CHAPTER TWO   34

INGREDIENTS TO A HEALTHY AND WELLNESS LIFE   34

WHAT ARE THE INGREDIENTS?   35

PRE-BIOTICS ESSENTIAL FOR HEALTH AND WELL-BEING   45

Health and Wellness in Drinking   47

Health and Wellness in Exercise   52

Sunshine, Free of Charge   57

Temperance   57

Skin Care Routine   58

Practice Contentment   58

CONCLUSION   62

CHAPTER ONE

INTRODUCTION TO HEALTH AND WELLNESS

WHAT IS HEALTH AND WELLNESS?

So much emphasis is placed on health and wellness these days it seems everywhere you turn you see or hear something about one or both of them. Have you ever considered what the terms health and wellness mean? Health, as defined by the World Health Organization (WHO) is a state of complete physical, mental and social well-being and not merely the absence of disease or infirmity (abnormal condition). This is only one attempt to define health. There are as many definitions of health as there are people because most people seem to perceive health in terms of their own ability to function according to their own perception of what is normal. Now that we know what health means, let's take a look at the definition of wellness.

Wellness can be defined as a state in which an individual of a given sex and at a given stage of growth and development is capable of meeting the minimum physical, physiological, and social requirements for appropriate functioning in the given sex category and at the given growth and developmental level. Another definition of wellness is a dynamic state of health in which an individual progresses toward a higher level of functioning, achieving an optimum balance between internal and external environments.

The term wellness can easily be divided into seven categories or dimensions; however, for the sake of this piece, we will concentrate on what I believe to be the top four.

•	Emotional Wellness: Being able to understand oneself and cope with life's challenges and its transitions without breaking down is emotional wellness. But it does not end there. It is the ability to share feelings in a productive manner. It's not just handling or managing stress but involves being connected to your thoughts, feelings and behaviors. And while many individuals have no disconnect with physical wellness, recognizing and understanding your true state of emotional wellness is still a delicate and unapproachable subject for many. However, in order to achieve optimum health, the state of your emotions must be explored and embraced.

•	Intellectual Wellness: Intellectual Wellness or mind wellness does not mean you are incredibly smart or free from psychosis or mental illness, but incorporates the desire to learn new ideas, experiences and concepts. It pursues lifelong learning not just about the outside world, but learning about yourself digging deep, if necessary, and connecting. Mind wellness invites you to explore and stretch. It challenges you to become mentally alert receiving all the signs sent by the brain. It demands being opened: stimulated by teachers, mentors, and personal guides. It is understanding and knowing the mind is where the healthy you dwells. While this area of wellness is the least popular, individuals are moving toward mindfulness theories finding their personal power.

•	Spiritual Wellness: There is an awakening happening throughout the world. People are understanding there is a shift occurring-a slow conscious shift toward understanding our planet and our surroundings. We are realizing there is something we all long and want to fulfil. Baby boomers, especially, are realizing a healthy soul equals a healthy body; the two are not separate. When you are spiritually awakened realizing you are one with yourself; you are in complete control of your life; and comprehend being the only authority in your life, you'll be willing to transcend questioning your true purpose, passion, and calling in life. This may seem a little hippy, but it works.

•	Physical Wellness: This dimension of wellness is the easiest to comprehend and more easily embraced. Physical wellness is the ability to maintain a healthy quality of life allowing you to get through your daily activities without undue fatigue or physical stress. It is taking responsibility for your physical duress. This may be accomplished by minor exercise or by pushing your body to physical extremes.
It includes building muscular strength and endurance, cardiovascular strength, flexibility, endurance and spiritual awakening. Optimal physical wellness is developed through the combination of physical activity and a healthy lifestyle. And, yes, that includes spirituality.

Interesting enough when you embrace the three dimensions of wellness mentioned previously, the physical stuff is easy. You'll have a strong desire to take personal responsibility for your healthcare understanding your body, knowing exactly what good health is for you.

Mentally alert and attuned, you'll know when serious medical attention is necessary, and you'll be comfortable in taking the appropriate action and making the right decision for yourself.

From the definitions of health and wellness, it is easy to see why a health history is requested when you see your physician or other health care professionals. Information requested may include your health history, family health history, diet, and exercise. Depending on the health care professional you are seeing, other information may be requested. Why is such a comprehensive history important to your physician or other health care professional? History provided by you gives your doctor or health care professional the most important tool to diagnose your condition and provide you with proper treatment. In other words, when you provide an honest and complete health history, family history, medical history, diet and exercise information you provide your doctor or health care professional insight regarding your health and wellness. Societal values also influence how an individual feels about maintaining a certain level of health.

To summarize, health means many things. It is a sense of complete well-being and the absence of disease. Each person's health falls somewhere on a line between the extremes of good health and illness. For the individual, the existence or absence of health is usually not determined solely by laboratory test or medical pronouncements but also by the expectations created within his/her particular society.

"If you have your health, you have everything," people say to one another and generally they understand what is meant.

IMPORTANCE OF HEALTH AND WELLNESS

The importance of health and wellness is significant in everyday life. There are primary components of health and fitness and secondary components. Primary components of health-related fitness consist of four main topics, which include: cardiorespiratory capacity, muscular capacity, flexibility, and body composition. Each part affects different aspects of health, fitness and wellness. Secondary components of fitness include seven different types of performance-based fitness, which are necessary for daily functioning and incorporated in all physical activity.

Health and wellness fit together but are also very different. Health is included in every human being and is constantly changing over time. Health can be considered good or bad, depending on whether or not a person is sick with an illness, cold, or contains bacteria. Health is also broken up into four separate types involving social health, mental health, emotional health, and spiritual health. Wellness, however, can depend on the person. Some people have the drive to obtain wellness in their daily life. Wellness is determined by a person's own responsibility on living out a healthy lifestyle.

There are numerous benefits you can get out of living a healthy lifestyle. It helps you achieve a healthy body and a revitalized mind. Here are some health benefits:

Health and wellness help increase your metabolism. If you have a good metabolism, you do not have to limit yourself from eating. You do not have to hunger your body just to achieve a healthy and sexy body. By increasing your metabolism, you can have a more natural way of burning up food and calories that you eat.

So you don't have to worry on how much food you wanted to eat because your metabolism will do the work for you. But then, it is still necessary to eat more healthy food rather than eating oily and saturated fatty foods.

Being healthy does not only make you feel good and healthy inside but it also makes your physical appearance look great and younger. When you feel old, you are most likely feel tired and restless so it means that your body is not in good shape. Now if you feel younger, you are more energetic to move and do all your tasks. If you are feeling young, it also affects the ageing process of your body and it certainly reflects your appearance. Feeling great just means looking fabulous.

Health and wellness programs such as physical activity also play a vital role in having a healthy mind and body. By regular exercise, you will be able to burn more calories and help you achieve the sexy body that you desire. This also prevents the development of any kinds of diseases such as heart problems, diabetes, high blood pressure and cancer. Health can be considered as our wealth because we only have one life to live. If we don't take good care of our health, most probably we'll have a shorter life to live.

Health and wellness should also involve avoiding or stopping bad habits like smoking, drinking alcohol and eating dangerous foods that can cause illness. As we all know, smoking is very dangerous to our health because it greatly affects the respiratory system and cardiovascular system. This eventually leads to lung cancer. Excessive drinking of alcohol can also cause a variety of health problems, it can severely damage your kidneys if you have too much of this. And of course, avoid eating foods that can cause diseases but instead eat more healthy food such as fruits and vegetables.

FOUR PILLARS OF HEALTH AND WELLNESS

Today's health care system, unfortunately, appears to be developing a generation of people who continue to stay sick and dependent on dangerous prescription drugs as plasters to the many symptoms of their sickness and diseases. Several studies have shown that these plasters are only known to weaken the immune system, the bio-energetic field and the critical pH balance of the human body.

Being Healthy will forever determine the longevity and quality of the life you live. But unfortunately most people today are either confused, or are purposely mislead into a variety of unhealthy habits and diet and may even be deceived about the natural healing powers of their amazing healing body, and what must be done to protect their 4 pillars of health.

1st Pillar of Health:
The 1st pillar of health which is tremendously critical to our health and wellness is our external bio-energetic field or our aura. This energy is like nothing else, you will feel pumped and ready for life. Basically, you will feel happy.

As the computer age continues to quickly move forward with the bombardment of electronic computers, gadgets, cell phones, iPhones, and several variations of electronic toys, studies have indicated that our aura of magnetic external protection continues to weaken thus allowing foreign elements to constantly attack and penetrate our body. In order to continue being healthy always, we must find ways to strengthen and protect this natural external defence to maintain our 4 pillars of health.

2nd Pillar of Health:
The 2nd pillar of health is our natural internal defence known as our immune system. The immune system was created to naturally protect the body from all diseases, and foreign invaders which enters our body, and which can seriously affect our health and wellness in our quest to being healthy always.

The great irony with respect to our immune system and the sick care system which pretends to function as our health care system is that the accepted methods of sick care treatment which is being touted, actually does more harm to our natural immune system, than actually doing any good.

Our immune system is made up of a number of stages and protective defensive agents. Some of these agents range from T-cells to B-cells, to Killer cells, to TH1 cells, to TH2 cells, to Cytotoxic T cells, and to Suppressor T cells, just to name a few. All of which were naturally created to ensure that the human body remains in a state of health and wellness by enhancing our 4 pillars of health. Confused don't panic it gets easier.

3rd Pillar of Health:
The 3rd pillar of health and wellness is our body pH balance. Being health simply means that your body pH balance is at an alkaline level of 7.356 of higher, as opposed to being at a pH balance level below 7 where all sick or diseased bodies are known to reside. The lower the body's pH balance level, the more acidic it is, and the greater the chances of that body being diseased.
The natural state of our body's pH balance is that of alkaline in the range of 7.356. From birth, our pH balance range is that of alkaline. But as we move forward into a polluted environment, including the processed and overcooked foods we constantly consume on a daily basis, together with the highly acidic beverages we consume, our body's pH balance gradually regresses into a state of acidity and eventual sickness.

4th Pillar of Health:

The 4th pillar of Health towards being healthy is our lifestyle. We need to have a system of regular exercise, daily preferably, but not necessarily vigorous. We need to reduce our intake of pollution from stress, toxins, carcinogens, and any other drugs or chemicals which may compromise our immune system.

The above 4 pillars of health have always proven to be vital in maintaining the perfect health and wellness of the body. We must find natural and positive ways of protecting our body from the outside to the inside.

Our amazing bio-energetic field or aura is constantly being bombarded as we sit in front of the many computers we constantly use. We cannot help but consume the right foods to not only prevent the imbalance of our body's pH balance, but we must also understand the dire need to protect our immune system by limiting or eliminating the use of carcinogens, of all forms, in our quest to being healthy, by protecting our 4 pillars of health.

SETTING GOALS TO ACHIEVE IMPROVED HEALTH AND WELLNESS

Now that the importance of health and wellness is understood by you. However, it can be difficult to make comprehensive changes in one's life that will result in optimal wellness. Setting goals and making incremental adjustments is often the best way to produce changes that will truly transform your life.

To begin making positive changes in your life, it is first important to have a strong desire for better health. This desire should come from within and should not be based on fear. A strong, positive desire to be healthier will provide the motivation needed to make positive changes.

Use the skills that coach's use and coach yourself to success. All you have to do is to be willing and committed to change. There is no secret.

Step 1: Know What You Want

When you coach yourself to success you have to know what success is, otherwise, how will you know when you've got there? This means that you have to know what you want to change and what the end result should look like.

If you already know what you want to change, but not what you want instead, you can come up with a statement of what you want by taking the opposite of what you don't want. If you don't want to weigh 200 pounds, how much do you want to weigh? If you don't want to work as a carpenter any longer, what do you want to work at?
The first question is easily answered and would lead you to focus on your desired weight. If you don't know the answer to the question, for example, you don't know what line of work you want, and then your focus would be on finding out the answer. You would first coach yourself to successfully find out what work would bring you joy, then coach yourself to find a job in that area.
If you don't know exactly where in your life you want to change, start with a wellness health assessment using a wheel of life. Draw a big circle, and divide it into segments and label them. Generally, wellness coaches use seven segments - physical body, mind, spirit, emotions, relationships, vocation/career, and environment. If you were to coach yourself to success at work, you would choose different labels.

For each segment in the wellness health assessment ask yourself on a scale of one to 10, where one represents no health and wellness and 10 represents complete health and wellness, how fulfilled and happy you feel in that area. Then, imagine that the centre of the circle is at one and the rim at 10 and .place a line across the segment (parallel to the rim) at the level of happiness you feel. Ask yourself what life would look like if you were at 10. For future reference, you can make a few notes inside the circle on what your life is like now for that segment, and outside the circle for what it would look like at a 10. Repeat for every segment.

Step 2: Choose One Thing to Change
It's important to take baby steps as you coach yourself to success. Don't try and change everything at once or you will likely become discouraged and give up. You might choose to work in an area you are particularly dissatisfied with or one where only a small change needs to be made.

Step 3: Set a Goal
To coach yourself to success, you must know what you want and keep the focus there, rather than on what you don't want. Goals focus you on the desired end result and keep you moving in the right direction. Your overall goal is to achieve health and wellness, but getting there will require many smaller specific goals.

Goals should be SMART - specific, measurable, actionable, realistic and timely. For example, 'I will weigh 120 pounds by September 1st 2020' meets these criteria, provided it would be possible to achieve that weight by then. It's often a good idea to set several short-term goals rather than one very long-term one, so you can monitor your progress and keep your spirits up. For the first month or so as you coach yourself to success you should have a goal for every week so that you start to feel successful.

Step 4: Take Action in Baby Steps
Choose one action that will move you towards the goal, and raise your fulfilment level in that health and wellness assessment area by just one point. Preferably choose something that must be done every day or more often. Repetition for 21 to 30 days develops a habit, and habits make actions effortless.
Step 5: Find a Structure
In coaching, structures are things that remind you to act. For example, setting an alarm clock is a structure that reminds you to get up early. Find something that will remind you to do the action you have chosen. You could set a schedule on your cell phone, or send yourself an email.

Step 6: Evaluate Regularly
Once a week hold a coach yourself to success meeting with yourself. Did you meet the goal or carry out the planned actions? If yes, celebrate! Then set another goal and another small action for the coming week while continuing with last week's action if that is appropriate.
If no, then beating yourself up is not in order - instead, find out what went wrong. Coaches ask their clients powerful questions that have no right or wrong answer, but which lead the client to explore themselves. As your own coach yourself to success coach, ask yourself questions like what got in the way of me doing what I had planned? How will I do it differently next week? Be curious and gentle with yourself. Set yourself a goal for the coming week that you think you can meet.

LAW OF ATTRACTION- HOW THE LAW OF ATTRACTION SUPPORTS HEALTH AND WELLNESS

We create all our situations, including social, financial and health in partnership with the Creator/Divinity/Source/Universe. Perhaps our thoughts got us into an accident, and then it created the result of the accident. This is why some people walk away from accidents unharmed that put others in the hospital. They use the Law of Attraction for health and well-being.

If you spend your youth worried that everyone in your family died from cancer, you are certainly going to attract cancer. It might not enter your life at 30 years of age, but at some point, it will because all that worry has to manifest the object of its worry. This is using the Law of Attraction for ill-health.

We also recreate the reality that we surround ourselves with. Business coaches will tell you that your income will be the average of the income of the five people closest to you. They encourage young business people to spend time with mentors and at conferences with those who have already achieved their goals because they see that this works. Those young people who move up the success ladder move faster when they have mentors and spend time with the already successful. This is also true of health.

Don't spend time with people who are doing everything wrong for their health. If you spend time at picnics and barbecues eating ribs and potato salad and drinking beer, you will see people gaining weight and hear about the health problems associated with their bad eating habits. Often those who eat badly also have bad activity habits or virtually no activity, and you will attract the things that they manifest because they will seem "normal" for your age group.

Spend time instead with those who are taking care of their physical well being if you want to improve your health. This is using the Law of Attraction for health. These people have the attitude of self-sufficiency and autonomy rather than an attitude of lack or helplessness and vulnerability. This doesn't have to be a $1200/year gym membership if you don't have the money or the time. It could be hiking outside the city on weekends, or taking a walk 5 times a week around a city park or both. Bicycling and rollerblading are great for your joint health if you come from a family that tends to develop arthritis.

People who are active might also develop influenza or even pneumonia, but because their bodies are more efficient, they will fight off these diseases more quickly and take less time to recover their energy and strength afterwards.

Use The Law Of Attraction For Health: Learn to Create the Emotion of Ease, and You Will Not Suffer from Dis-ease:

Spend time basking in the appreciation for your wellness. Spend time with good thoughts about your comfort and stamina and you will only lose them for brief periods of time. Good feelings product good health and well being. This is the law of vibrations.

Most disease today is not from any pathogen that entered our bodies from the outside, but from internal distress that interferes with or interrupts our normal and healthy systems. Dr Bruce Lipton talks about your intelligent cells. They each know what they need for health and vitality and they move toward those good things and move away from those things that are toxic and bad for them. But, if you provide them with a toxic environment, they will not be able to move far enough away. He first discovered this when he took cancerous, tumor cells from the body and grew them in a petri dish. He found that they began to behave normally once they were again in a normal, healthy enough environment.

What? Yes, cancer cells are not sick cells, but normal cells that are in a sick environment. So, it is your job to create as loving and harmonious an environment as possible. If you do this, your cells will be happy and your health will be continuous and steady. This is the Law of Attraction for health.

Searching for What's Wrong will Create Illness or Disability:

Those who go to the doctor looking for the problem will create a problem. This is the Law of Attraction at work. And, most doctors will find a problem eventually if you give them, and your ability to manifest, enough time. They will take tests and give you ideas of "What might be wrong" and eventually, one will stick.

The Law of Attraction insists on this. It is not that there was something there at the beginning, but if you continuously look for it, and think about it, it will manifest.

So work to deliberately manifest well being and health. You might be inspired to be more active. Don't ignore inspiration, but don't worry about it either. Take it as inspiration to improve your health and well being rather than to correct a problem.

Your health is profoundly affected by your beliefs. I have watched many friends get older, while I stay able to get into shape and to do whatever I ask my body to do. Sometimes I suffer afterwards if I push harder than usual, but we always re-establish equilibrium at a more efficient level after a crisis, so this is a good thing.

This is not to say that going to a doctor is necessarily a bad thing. If you are inspired to go to the doctor, go, but go with a sense of your body's ability to heal itself and with a sense of your well-being. This is the way to go into any test. This is the Law of Attraction at work showing itself in your health.

Accept Instead, the Stream of Well-Being:

The sense of well-being is a stream that flows continuously from Source energy/Universe/Divinity/your beliefs to us. It is only stopped by our own resistance. If we practice being in a state of allowing, we will always experience health through the Law of Attraction.

Any illness is an example of resistance. Bill Harris explains this in his training, it helps to remove resistance as they increase the good kind of stress that will raise your ability to deal with stress. Some people experience pain during this. He gives clear and detailed instructions as to how you can let go of resistance by being in the pain and accepting the pain. It is almost miraculous that as soon as you notice pain, and accept it, it diminishes and disappears.

Use the Law of Attraction for Wealth-

Remember the Law of Attraction can be applied to just about any aspect of your life. Here though I want to touch upon how it influences our wealth. No doubt you've heard the saying "the rich get richer whilst the poor get poorer", this is actually based on truth and although primarily based on the privatized banking system which lends money at the interest it's also very closely related to the Law of Attraction!

You see the thing is whilst the central banking system is responsible for such a divide among the rich and poor on a large commercial-scale, how "rich" we become as individuals is by our own choosing. As the Law of Abundance states; you can have anything you want out of life.

Rich people have a positive attitude and certain philosophies towards wealth and financial success, they understand money invested wisely makes more money, they also understand that by believing in themselves and maintaining a positive attitude they will naturally become richer in so many ways.

The problem for people experiencing financial difficulties is that they focus all their thoughts and mental energy into never having enough money and being poor. This negative attitude and negative thought patterns will only dampen their manifestation efforts and slow down the process of them receiving that which they desire, which of course is to be financially free.

To sum up it's worth noting that the Law of Attraction is always at work whether you're aware of it or not. The key for harnessing the power of this universal law lays within your attitude and thoughts. Focus on remaining positive, if something feels good then keep on doing it, take whatever steps you can further boost your manifestation efforts.

Remember the Law of Attraction can be applied to just about any aspect of your life. Here though I want to touch upon how it influences our wealth. No doubt you've heard the saying "the rich get richer whilst the poor get poorer", this is actually based on truth and although primarily based on the privatized banking system which lends money at interest it's also very closely related to the Law of Attraction!

You see the thing is whilst the central banking system is responsible for such a divide among the rich and poor on a large commercial-scale, how "rich" we become as individuals is by our own choosing. As the Law of Abundance states; you can have anything you want out of life.

Rich people have a positive attitude and certain philosophies towards wealth and financial success, they understand money invested wisely makes more money, they also understand that by believing in themselves and maintaining a positive attitude they will naturally become richer in so many ways.

The problem for people experiencing financial difficulties is that they focus all their thoughts and mental energy into never having enough money and being poor. This negative attitude and negative thought patterns will only dampen their manifestation efforts and slow down the process of them receiving that which they desire, which of course is to be financially free.

To sum up it's worth noting that the Law of Attraction is always at work whether you're aware of it or not. The key for harnessing the power of this universal law lays within your attitude and thoughts. Focus on remaining positive, if something feels good then keep on doing it, take whatever steps you can further boost your manifestation efforts.

Rule # 1: More Is More.

In this case, the more you think about it, the more of it you'll get. Money-wise, it can be anything from more money to more debt. For your sake, I hope that you're thinking of accumulating assets rather than liabilities.

Of course, when you're knee-deep in loans, it's hard to think of anything else but your problems. But remember, it only takes one thought to turn your life around. Make that thought a positive one.

Rule # 2: Green Light Goals.

To make full use of the law of attraction for wealth, it needs to lead up to something. Whether it's a savings account worth six figures or a trip of a lifetime, you must have a goal to keep you going.

In fact, many companies are now encouraging their employees to make vision boards to remind them of what is at stake. Wherever the vision is, prosperity follows.

If you try using the law of attraction to manifest abundance without a specific goal, the whole exercise becomes pointless.

Rule # 3: Adopt An Attitude Of Gratitude.

Using the law of attraction for wealth is also heavily rooted in gratitude. Whether you have received what you asked for or not, you must adopt an attitude of appreciation. After all, it is often said that success is 80% attitude and 20% aptitude.

When it comes to settling your finances, the same belief holds true. Having a good attitude about money increases your chances of attracting it in your life.

One way you can focus your energies into that of appreciation is by starting a gratitude list. Every day, list down whatever you are grateful for. As the days go by, you'll find yourself having more and more to add to the list.

Using the law of attraction for wealth can produce powerful results. However, it is also important to note that wealth is not just about cold, hard cash. It's also about having fruitful connections and meaningful relationships.

CHAPTER TWO

INGREDIENTS TO A HEALTHY AND WELLNESS LIFE

WHAT ARE THE INGREDIENTS?

We hear so much about the importance of our diet when it comes to health. I would like to suggest to you that there are several aspects to our health that can be achieved and maintained beyond what we eat. I invite you to take a look at the following as we discuss recipes and health in a very different way.

When we think about health the thought that most of us have begins and ends with what we eat. Yet what if what we can learn about health isn't limited to food? You see the reason diets work is that at the end of the day a diet is a mathematical problem put on paper. It is calories in versus calories out. When we cook from home we use these healthy recipes and if we stick with them religiously we see success.

Taking things a step further what if we applied the same system to other aspects of our health and wellness. Why don't we have a recipe for sleep, a recipe for stress management, a recipe for stretching, a recipe for exercise and a recipe for relaxation? Recipes are nothing more than a written plan of preparing to cook. Some may be passed down for generations at home and some are used in restaurants. Some are original and some may be copied. The recipe for Cola has often been attempted to be copied yet continues to be kept well protected over the years. Remember when Cola tried to discontinue its product and introduced New Cola? It became one of the biggest advertising mistakes of the last century and a lesson that can apply in both business and in health, "if it ain't broke don't fix it."

The fact is that while diets do work and of course our food choices do matter, I subscribe to you that the reason perhaps that we have more success with food than we do with other health challenges is that we normally have a plan when it comes to food. Yet with exercise, stress, sleep and a variety of other related subjects we seemingly try to go with the flow and just wing it.

It is important to note that we can learn much from the process of creating a recipe. Recipes create consistency, reliability and predictability. A written plan of attack if you will for the foods we eat. So let's have a written plan when it comes to other aspects of our health and well-being. Let me take you through simple tips to get better results fast on your health and wellness journey.

Health and Wellness in Eating

For the body to remain in a state of health and balance, attention must be paid daily to the concept of eating for health as well as eating for pleasure. In this section, you will learn how super foods and super supplements can change the biochemistry of the body. They help reverse stress patterns, disease patterns, that when left unchecked, cause many types of illness, such as high blood pressure, high cholesterol, heart disease, chronic pain, premature ageing of all body organs and many other common symptoms.

What Are Super Foods And Why Are They Considered Super?

Super Foods are foods that are found to produce certain types of positive biochemical changes in the body and contain nutrients known to have medicinal properties. The biochemical changes can repair, heal, and restore the body back to health and balance by repairing damaged cellular tissue, and bone. Studies by many medical universities have found that the active phytonutrients in superfoods help to cure and prevent symptoms.

The Top 10 Super foods are:
i.   Acai berry,
ii.   The allium family (onion, garlic, shallots, leeks, scallions),
iii.   Barley,
iv.   Beans,
v.   Lentils, buckwheat,
vi.   All green vegetables,
vii.   Hot peppers,
viii.   Nuts and seeds,
ix.   Sprouts and yoghurt. These foods should be staples in the daily diet.

What are Super Supplements?
Super supplements can be described as the active ingredient in a highly nutritional food. When concentrated, and taken in high doses it produces a medicinal effect. The most important supplements are: amino acids, antioxidants, acidophilus, berry and green plant concentrates. When these substances are added to a clean healthy diet and lifestyle, your overall health, energy, stamina, and brain chemistry are given the extra nutrients that are needed. They give your body optimum energy and performance, as well as changing and reversing disease patterns.

- Antioxidants
Antioxidants reverse free radical damage to tissue caused by chemicals and environmental toxins. They also encourage natural digestive enzymes that help proper colon functioning. Antioxidants promote proper blood ph levels, which help to stop inflammation in all body tissue and joints. The most famous antioxidants are fruit and green vegetable concentrates, wheat and barley grasses. The fruits and berries include acai, blueberries, cranberries, goji berries, pomegranate, and mangosteen. Wheat, barley, and oat grass are also famous for their detoxifying properties. They have been used in the Middle East and the Orient for thousands of years and are considered blood and energy tonics.

- Amino Acids

Amino acids are the individual organic chemicals that are in proteins and can be found in Whey Powder products. Amino acids considered the building blocks for all cells. All muscle and brain tissue are fed by amino acids. They help in tissue repair, create antibodies that fight bacteria and viruses, enhance energy, fight fatigue, and stabilize blood sugar. They are famous for enhancing muscle mass and strength. Certain amino acids repair DNA damage from environmental toxins and chemical toxins from food. Individual amino acid supplements, such as Taurine can be effective in high doses to calm the nervous system. Tyrosene in high doses can stimulate the thyroid and brain neurotransmitters that increase energy and metabolism. Amino acids and amino acid deficiencies can be tested with very sophisticated testing, taking the guesswork out of what the body needs.

- Acidophilus

Acidophilus are called "good guy" intestinal bacteria. They help to keep the natural flora of the intestines and vagina balanced. These bacteria are of critical importance for all breakdown and metabolism of food. Just increasing acidophilus levels into normal ranges cure many gastrointestinal problems. They also help protect the body by fighting against invasion of harmful bacteria, parasites, and other organisms. Acidophilus is also involved in all vitamin synthesis, natural antibiotic production, immune defence, and detoxification of pro-carcinogens and a host of other activities. Acidophilus is naturally occurring in yoghurt but for medicinal purposes, it should be taken in high dose supplementation.

- Essential Fatty Acids
These are the fats the body cannot make and therefore must be added to the diet.
These essential fatty acids are widely distributed in plant and fish oils. Primarily used to produce hormone-like substances that regulate a wide range of things including, proper brain functioning, dropping blood pressure, helping blood clotting, controlling lipid levels, supporting immune response, and all inflammatory responses. Essential Fatty Acids are comprised of two groups: Omega 3 and Omega 6 and 9. These oils need to be supplemented on a daily basis, as the body cannot make them. Using cold pressed organic oils from nuts, seeds, and vegetables are good daily routines. All oils can be taken in pill form or liquid form and high doses are recommended for certain illnesses.

The body has an amazing capability to heal and continually restore itself, given the right environment. Every day we can change our biochemistry positively or negatively, by the foods and supplements that we take in. To be able to live healthy, active lives, we must take very good care of our bodies, and make healthy choices. Not only will this benefit us by feeling better immediately, but it will help stop disease and prevent chronic illness and premature ageing.

We need to start thinking that eating for health can be a great source of pleasure. Antioxidants, acidophilus, essential oils, and amino acids are the " Super Supplements" that become an added bonus of ensuring optimum health, energy, and vitality.

The easy way to get all the nutrition required is to eat a well-balanced diet. This will maintain a healthy body. Eating plenty of vegetables, legumes and fruit is an essential part of a healthy diet, as is eating cereals including grains, pasta, bread (preferably wholegrain). The consumption of lean meat, fish and poultry are desirable, this is what our not so distant ancestors consumed on a daily basis. Vegetarians can make alternative arrangements to provide their protein requirements. The consumption of dairy products is fine. There is debate as to whether the levels of saturated fats in dairy are actually bad for you, moderation is the key, but if you feel concerned about saturated fats, then consider low-fat products.

Macro-nutrients

The essential macro-nutrients of carbohydrate, protein and fats are essential for health and well-being. How do we decide how much nutrient is required to prevent deficiencies? The National Academy of Sciences makes these recommendations.

Protein: 10-35% Fat: 20-35% Carbohydrate:45-65%
Eating the correct quantities of these macro-nutrients can help in reducing the risk of chronic diseases, whilst providing all the essential vitamins, minerals and nutrients we require. A healthy lifestyle can be achieved by regular exercise and a balanced diet with correct quantities of macro and micronutrients.
Let's look at the nutrients in functions of foods that might be beneficial...
Plant stanols and sterols - these substances are a natural part of fruits, veggies, nuts and seeds and chemically resemble cholesterol. But when they go through your digestive system, they block the real cholesterol and keep it from entering your bloodstream.
You should try to get 2 grams of plant stanols and sterols a day.

•   Vitamin D - together with calcium, helps bones stay strong and boosts the immune system. There's research that suggests this vitamin might also help prevent some cancers, hypertension and even depression. The trouble is most of us don't get nearly enough. Babies need 400 IU a day, kids between 1 and 16 need 800 IUs daily, adults between 19 to 70 should be aiming for 600 IUs and seniors should be getting 800 IUs of vitamin D a day.

With our diets, and indoor lifestyles (vitamin D is made naturally when we're exposed to sunlight), it's easy to see why we don't get enough.

Calcium - well known to help build bones; it also transmits nerve impulses to keep your heart pumping, though most of us don't get enough. If your body doesn't have the calcium it needs from foods, it may start to take the mineral from your bones, which can bring on osteoporosis.
Eating three portions of low-fat dairy each day should give you the amount of calcium your body needs. But if you're not a fan of dairy products, functional foods will make up the shortfall. One note, calcium that comes from fortified foods might not be as well absorbed by the body compared to foods where it occurs naturally.
Babies need 210-270 mg of calcium, and a kid under 8 needs 500-800 mg. After 9 a child's need for calcium jumps to 1,300 mg, while most adults should be getting 1,000 mg per day.

•   Fibre - is a type of carbohydrate that's naturally a part of plants and helps us to feel full, keeps our bowels working properly and might even bring down the chance of developing of heart disease or diabetes. Most people don't get enough according to the USDA guidelines. Women should be aiming for 25 grams a day; men 38 grams of fiber a day.
While most of our fiber should be supplied from whole foods like beans, veggies and whole grains, added fiber found in bread or cereal is a reasonable option, though it's not clear if this has the same benefit as if it came from the natural sources.

There are two types of fiber, soluble (beans and nuts) which slow digestion and insoluble (veggies and whole grains) that aids food in passing through your body.

•	Omega-3 Fatty Acids - include the DHA and EPA your body needs so that your brain works properly and nerves develop, while research suggests they might also be helpful in improving memory and your mood while cutting the chance of heart disease. While they are naturally a part of fish like salmon, cod, tuna and sardines, and in smaller amounts in seeds and nuts.

Omega-3s are commonly added to all kinds of functional foods, from eggs to cereal to soy, though the most frequently added one, ALA (alpha-linolenic acid) may not bring the same benefits to health as DHA or EPA does. Many functional foods just don't have enough omega-3, so it may be a good idea to take supplements to increase your levels.

PRE-BIOTICS ESSENTIAL FOR HEALTH AND WELL-BEING

Prebiotics are components present in foods, or that can be incorporated into foods, which give health by supporting the gastrointestinal tract (GI) by giving the body what it needs to defend itself.

Pre-biotics are a type of fiber which can help protect the body against food poisoning, intestinal and colon problems. Most importantly, pre-biotics are food for our "good" gut bacteria. As a result, they promote the growth of these healthy bacteria and help inhibit the overgrowth of pathogenic ones.

Typically, prebiotics are carbohydrates, but the definition does not preclude non-carbohydrates. The most prevalent forms of pre-biotics are nutritionally classed as soluble fiber. To some extent, many forms of dietary fiber exhibit some level of pre-biotic effect.

A pre-biotic should increase the number of bifid bacteria and lactic acid bacteria, and can also make them more powerful and active. The importance of the bifid bacteria and the lactic acid bacteria is that they benefit people by improving digestion, increasing absorption and boosting immune system.

Today, probiotic-containing foods are commonly found and consumed. Pre-biotic are found naturally in many foods, and can also be isolated from plants. In order for a food ingredient to be classified as a prebiotic, it has to be demonstrated that it is not broken down in the stomach or absorbed in the GI tract, and that it is fermented by the gastrointestinal micro flora. It must also stimulate the growth and activity of intestinal bacteria associated with health and well-being.

This pre-biotic fibre is found primarily in certain vegetables listed below:

- Chicory Root
- Jerusalem Artichoke
- Leeks
- Onions
- Salsify
- Bananas
- Oats

You may benefit from eating pre-biotic if you:

- Have a blood sugar imbalance- pre-biotic encourage bifid bacteria to grow which produce acids which help balance blood sugar levels
- Are prone to stomach upsets or gut dysbiosis
- Are travelling to areas where gastrointestinal illness is common
- Suffer from gastroenteritis, Crohn's disease or ulcerative colitis
- If you are taking antibiotics
- Are prone to thrush or bacterial vaginosis

Make sure your vegetables are as fresh as possible as long storage times lowers their nutrient and pre-biotic content

Onion soup is one of the best ways to obtain a large dose of pre-biotics and it is one of the highest natural sources of vitamin C

Some people may get excessive flatulence eating these foods. Simply start on a very low dosage per day and build up gently. Eventually, the good bacteria will build up in the gut and the flatulence will cease. Anyone with arthritis or other auto-immune conditions should use pre-biotics with caution.

Health and Wellness in Drinking

Your body needs water to hydrate cells and flush out toxins. Several daily ailments like low energy, headaches and constipation will improve greatly if you just increase your water intake. Remember I did not say your fluid intake. Coffee and pop have no nutritional value and will not hydrate you.

How Much Water Do We Really Need?
The average 150-pound adult is made up of approximately 2/3rds water. That's 40-50 quarts of water or 80-100 pounds of water per person! Our bodies use about three quarts of water a day to carry out its normal functions. That water needs to be replaced with additional water and through the foods, we eat.

Many experts agree that most normally active, healthy people do best when they drink about a ½ ounce of water per pound of bodyweight. That's roughly eight to ten cups of water daily.

Caffeinated beverages do provide water but the caffeine causes the body to release water so these drinks are poor choices for hydration. If you don't like the taste of plain water, squeeze in some fresh lemon or lime juice. An easy way to determine if you are drinking enough water is that you do not feel thirsty and your urine is light yellow to clear in colour.

Water is necessary for the proper functioning of all organs and systems in the body. All parts of your body are made up of varying amounts of water. You need it to properly digest your food, absorb nutrients, remove toxins and eliminate waste from the body. It improves mental and physical performance. Even mild dehydration can increase your chances of developing a headache, viral infection, heart attack or kidney stones. Blood becomes thicker and harder to circulate, creating a feeling of brain fog and tiredness.

Tips for Drinking Water

•	Have a glass or two of water as soon as you get up in the morning and before bed. Keep a glass of water by your bed if you get thirsty during the night. Don't worry, your bladder will adjust.

•	Cold water will help you cool off and temporarily speed up your metabolism. This can help you burn calories.

•	If you feel cold, drink warm water with lemon or have a dilute non-caffeinated drink.

•	Keep a source of water with you at all times. Refillable water bottles with a built-in filter can be filled at any faucet and have the added benefit of reducing the expense and waste generated by pre-filled water bottles.

•	Have a glass of water a few minutes before your meal to reduce feelings of hunger and provide water to aid the digestion process. If you are in the habit of drinking at mealtime, take small sips. Too much water while eating can interfere with digestion.

•	If you feel hungry between meals, take a moment and ask yourself, "Am I really hungry or am I thirsty?" Often you will find that you are really thirsty. This can help you cut back on excessive calories.

•	Increase your water consumption when you are very active, if you are taking diuretics, or drinking alcohol and caffeinated drinks.
Note: Some health conditions may require you to monitor your water consumption. Please consult a physician before making changes to your health regimen.

Juicing for Health and Wellness

Health experts agree that to protect ourselves from illness and disease and to enjoy optimum health, we should eat more fruits and vegetables and what better way to add them to our diets than juicing. The chemicals in plants, phytochemicals, protect the body from many forms of cancer, as well as heart disease and many age-related diseases like arthritis. Juicing with fresh fruits and veggies gives your body phytochemicals, nutrients and enzymes in an easily digestible form so your body can absorb them quickly and with maximum benefits.

- Juicing Provides A Meal In A Glass

How does juicing deliver the best nutrition? To make one glass of carrot juice, for instance, it takes a pound of carrots. What better way to consume that many carrots in a day than by juicing? It takes little or no digestive effort to assimilate juiced foods directly into the body so all those healing; healthful nutrients find their way right into your bloodstream.

- Juicing Delivers Enzymes

There are 55,000 enzymes in the human body, divided into three different types.

Digestive enzymes are made by the body, such as the enzymes in saliva, to help digest food.

Food enzymes come from the raw food we eat, such as fresh fruits and vegetables. Heating food to a temperature of 114 degrees F destroys these enzymes. If you eat only cooked food, you aren't getting the enzymes necessary to the proper functioning of the body at the cellular level.

Metabolic enzymes enable the proper functioning of the body and provide regeneration and energy at the cellular level.
The use of fresh, raw fruits and vegetables through juicing makes this drink powerhouse of enzymes which then play an essential role in protecting cells from damage.

- Juicing Delivers Nutrients

Fruits and vegetables are also excellent sources of other essential vitamins and minerals. Juicing breaks them down into a liquid form more easily absorbed by the body. The fiber in whole fruit and vegetables, removed through juicing, traps the nutrients so the body can't absorb them as easily. Through juicing nearly 100% of nutrients are absorbed by the body.

Juicing also delivers the natural water available in fresh fruits and vegetables to your body. Fruits and vegetables, like human bodies, are made up largely of water.

Health and Wellness in Exercise

The next component in health and wellness that people know about is exercise. Balancing the body does require the whole physical body, inside and out. Need to tighten the stomach muscles? See a 'love handle' that has multiplied? This is what many people see in the mirror and motivates them to lose weight. Exercising the body can assist in the improvement of organ functioning and the blood circulation in the body. I must, however, emphasize that not all exercise is created equal and that there are certainly efficient ways of exercising and also inefficient ways to exercise. Most people think that exercising with weights is the best way to get yourself into tip top shape, and while it may be true that exercising with weights is a great way to build muscle tone and definition, cardiovascular health may really be your first concern when exercising. The reason that some stress cardiovascular health over exercising with weights is because having a strong base of cardiovascular health may go a long way to improve all aspects of your physicality especially if you do begin to lift weights.

So, what are some general tips to get yourself started with an exercise program? The first thing that most would suggest doing is running or high paced walking. You don't necessarily have to start out running 5-minute miles and breaking national records, but running is perhaps the greatest exercise when developing cardiovascular fitness. If you find that you are unable to run for any appreciable amount of time than you can always start out walking on a fast pace that you can handle. Once you are able to increase your walking speed you can begin to run in intervals where you might run for 1 minute and walk for 2 minutes. You shouldn't be killing yourself during these interval runs, but rather you should be working just hard enough to tax your breathing.

The old wisdom goes that you should be able to talk while running, but you should not be able to carry on long sentences or sing. As you build up your endurance by practising intervals you will eventually want to work on the amount of distance you can run before having to stop. At first, it may be a half mile and then in another month and maybe a mile, but you always want to keep pushing yourself to go a little bit further.

Exercising with weights is also a great way to stay in shape, but as I stated earlier some find it to be a subordinate activity to running and other forms of cardiovascular exercise.

Exercising with weights can be as simple as purchasing a set of dumbbells and performing some routine chest, back, leg, and shoulder exercises. You don't need to go all out with the weights, but if you do decide that you would like to get more involved in this aspect of exercise, you might consider joining in a local gym to further your goals. The long and short of it is that any form of exercise is good so long as you practice good form, moderation, and work out intelligently. Stick to these principles and you will be the best shape of your life in no time.

Health and Wellness with Yoga
Though often described as an optional health branch, yoga is a science in itself with intricacies that only the advanced teachers can explain. Though you can find many yoga masters in the west, most are born and educated in India. There are varieties of techniques in yoga which are most suitable for your individual needs. These techniques differ for a woman, a teenager, an aged individual, a child and an athlete.
Yoga for health and wellness has several benefits and fulfils needs for nearly all individuals. It helps everyone to play their roles efficiently, smoothly and comfortably. Yoga compared with other exercises such as gymnastics and aerobics has several advantages. You can practice yoga inside your house or outside alone or in groups. It needs to be practiced on an empty stomach and can be performed any time during the day.

Yoga for health aid prevents diseases and illnesses and maintains health and fitness in your daily life. Though all age groups can practice yoga effectively, some techniques are appropriate for some age groups only. For instance, asanas which include forward, and backward bending are good for kids from 6 to 10 years.

Yoga for Health
Yoga, when practiced properly, has advantages of flexible joints, muscles, relaxed and tension free mind and effectively working vital organs such as heart, lungs, pancreas, liver and endocrine glands.
Yoga brings in wonderful changes that have a deep effect on the mental health of a person and these changes are reduction in tension and restoration of flexibility. Yoga also increases the capacity for alertness, attentiveness and motivation for tackling various problems. It also creates a powerful and positive connection between emotional and physical health.
There are specific health benefits associated with yoga which are unique and are beyond the advantages of any exercise program. It can be as energetic or as gentle as you need it to be. You can take help of a yoga instructor who can work with your individual fitness level for modifying various postures to suit you.

Yoga is one of several naturopathic approaches to enhance wellbeing and promote health. Iyengar yoga, in particular, focuses on healing. In this type, accurate application of alignment is used to free the body from the negative effects of poor alignment and improper posture. The instructors here use blocks, cushions, benches, straps and bean bags to make proper adjustments to the posture for absolute postural alignment.

You can maintain proper health and wellness by practicing various yoga exercises and postures regularly. Remember yoga complements other natural methods of healing for improving the energy flow throughout the body. Practicing different postures, therapeutic massage therapy etc. help ensure any minor discomforts are reconciled before they worsen and affect other areas of the body.

Sunshine, Free of Charge

Sunshine is known to be the best source of vitamin D. In addition to strengthening one's bones, Vitamins are antioxidants that are given credit for reversing as well as preventing most degenerative diseases such as cancer and the likes.

Temperance

Temperance is a virtue that is with only a small portion of the population. It means using the healthy substances in moderation were as completely discarding the unhealthy products. How many will say that "For sure, I know that carbonated drinks such as Cola aren't healthy for me but I can't stop using them?" that's intemperance.

Oxygen from Fresh Air

Fresh air is vital for proper respiration to take place. Cancer cells only survive where anaerobic respiration takes place. It is therefore important for you to exercise in places with fresh air so as to ensure all your body cells respire aerobically. When attending to a sick person, it's in order to take them to sanitariums that are located in areas with many trees for fresh air.

Skin Care Routine

Drink plenty of water; 8 glasses each day. Eat lots of yellow and orange fruits which provide Vitamin A. Take a good Vitamin E supplement. Eat cucumbers, which supply sulphur - a trace element that is necessary for healthy skin!! Also use water-based moisturizing creams or olive oil on the skin, immediately after bathing to keep moisture locked into your skin.

Practice Contentment

In the natural ebb and flow of life and living, there are high points and low points, seasons of plenty and seasons of scarcity. Happiness is not derived from the abundance, number or type of material things we have. That's why we sometimes see examples of millionaires who are drug addicts or alcoholics. Added to that, there is the "Law of Diminishing Returns". What this basically says is that the more we get of something up to a certain point, the less likely the added quantities of that thing is going to increase our happiness quota. It's like if I got one (1) Lamborghini - I am on a high, summersaults can't express my happiness, I could hug everybody I meet. If I got two (2) more Lamborghinis - well that's OK. I mean I really won't feel as euphoric as that first time and in any case, how many can I drive at any one time?

Contentment is the ability to be happy in both the sparse and abundant seasons of our lives and it is not dependent on our circumstances. We need to develop this spirit of contentment in order to positively contribute to our overall health, happiness and well-being. This does not mean that we should not strive for better but it means that like the old West Indian say goes, "We shouldn't hang our hats where our hands can't reach", in order to keep up with the Jones'.

Take the Care of Your Mind Seriously.
Stress and Depression are two (2) of the biggest thieves of mental and emotional health, globally. Not only are they globally prevalent but they also lead to more serious mental problems such as Dementia, Alzheimer's, Suicide and Insanity.
In fact, "The World Health Organization estimates that more than 450 million people [worldwide] suffer from mental disorders, and a new report by the World Economic Forum figures the annual global costs of mental and neurological illnesses at $2.5 trillion. That is three times the economic cost of heart disease 'Global mental health issues woefully overlooked', Public Radio International."

So stress and depression must be dealt with and arrested almost immediately in order to avoid more serious health problems. Depression is a natural phase that we all experience in our lives primarily due to loss of loved ones, work issues, job loss or money/financial issues. However, the key to ensuring that stress and depression do not get out of hand is engaging in activities that move your mind away from the problem causing the stress or depression and move you to a better mental space, despite the problem at hand. You can improve and maintain the health of your brain by incorporating some of these simple techniques into your daily living.

Simple Mental Health Care Solutions
•   Board Games, Puzzles & Quizzes
Playing Board Games and Solving Puzzles & Quizzes all provide your brain with a mental workout by improving your memory, concentration, problem-solving skills and preventing cognitive decline.

•   Listening to music
Although seemingly simple, music soothes the mind and spirit, helps the body relax, relieves mental and emotional stress and tension, stimulates the senses and energizes the body.

- Writing

There are many great online writing communities, such as EzineArticles and Squidoo, which accept articles on just about any topic that you would be interested in. Again, you will be exercising your brain, since to write an excellent article you will need to do some research to supplement your knowledge of the area.

- Hobbies and Sports

Engage in group activities, social clubs or sports that interest you (tennis, horse riding, soccer, football, cricket, karate, sewing, yoga, tai chi, basketball, volleyball, swimming, singing, dancing etc.). Anything that you are naturally inclined to and that makes you feel happy while doing it.

What about Rest?

Work without sufficient rest is one of the greatest forms of intemperance being suffered by humanity. Eight hours of sleep, most preferably starting at least two hours before midnight is recommended. In addition, a thirty-minute nap in the afternoon is therapeutic. Also, ensure that you take a day's rest every week.

CONCLUSION

Every living being sought optimal health and happiness, a quality of life where there is a healthy balance between the mind, body, soul and spirit. Our ultimate goal is to live a life of purpose, one of meaning, to love and to be loved, and be healthy. Life throws everything at you, and you frantically juggle to keep things balanced. The pieces come together to create our unique lives that are forever changing. With this comes a feeling of well-being, status of our wellness. It is the combination of the physical, mental, spiritual, intellectual, social, environmental and socioeconomic components that determines our overall state of health.

The abundance of information about health and wellness in this book is enough to take you through the journey of a fulfilling life.

Life is magnificent and we all deserve to enjoy it to its fullest. There are some things we cannot control but mostly we have the power to choose how to live and react. Taking small steps to introduce healthier habits will make a significant difference to your overall health, remembering to maintain constructive balance of all components. Don't wait until it's too late as some things are difficult to reverse.

Modern life can be stressful and leave you overwhelmed, this may lead to an unhealthy body and unsatisfied life.